MW00774465

To:

From:

FIRST AID
for the
SOUL at
CHRISTMAS

Compiled by Sonya V. Tinsley

Illustrated by Jane Heyes

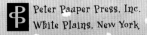

Peter Pauper Press, Inc.

White Plains, New York

Designed by Kerren Barbas

Illustrations copyright © 2000
Jane Heyes
Licensed by Wild Apple Licensing

Text copyright © 2000
Peter Pauper Press, Inc.
202 Mamaroneck Avenue
White Plains, NY 10601

Visit us at
www.peterpauper.com

FIRST AID
for the
SOUL at
CHRISTMAS

Introduction

There is a time for mirth and a time for madness—and it's called Christmas! Christmas creates such glorious contradictions. We are the faithful children waiting expectantly for the miracles we know are coming. We are the flustered grown-ups who fear *only* a miracle will help us make it through our holiday to-do lists.

This season, whether we are making wishes or frantically trying to fill them, the voices in this book will speak to our souls.

S. V. T.

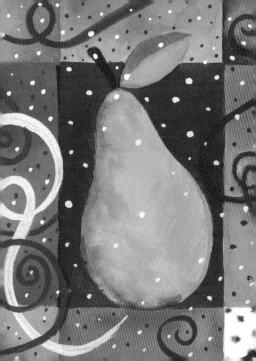

Christmas-time [is] the only time I know of, in the long calendar of the year, when men and women seem by one consent to open their shut-up hearts freely, and to think of people below them as if they really were fellow-passengers to the grave, and not another race of creatures bound on other journeys.

Charles Dickens, A Christmas Carol

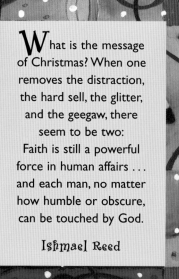

Whatisthemessage
of Christmas? When one
removes the distraction,
the hard sell, the glitter,
and the geegaw, there
seem to be two:
Faith is still a powerful
force in human affairs . . .
and each man, no matter
how humble or obscure,
can be touched by God.

Ishmael Reed

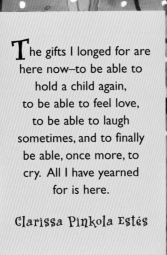

The gifts I longed for are
here now—to be able to
hold a child again,
to be able to feel love,
to be able to laugh
sometimes, and to finally
be able, once more, to
cry. All I have yearned
for is here.

Clarissa Pinkola Estés

Think about the things
you enjoy most in
life, and try to find a
way of incorporating
them as your own
holiday customs.

B. Smith

[A]t least for
a season, it seems
"peace on Earth,
goodwill toward men"
might be possible
after all.

Jeffrey L. Sheler

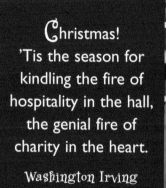

Christmas!
'Tis the season for
kindling the fire of
hospitality in the hall,
the genial fire of
charity in the heart.

Washington Irving

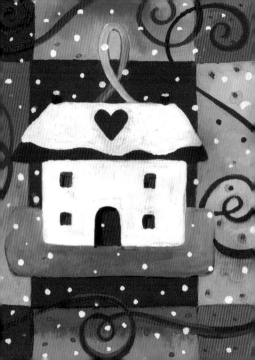

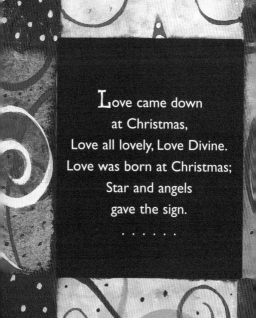

Love came down
at Christmas,
Love all lovely, Love Divine.
Love was born at Christmas;
Star and angels
gave the sign.

. . . . . .

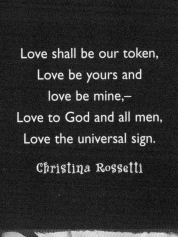

Love shall be our token,
Love be yours and
love be mine,–
Love to God and all men,
Love the universal sign.

Christina Rossetti

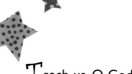

Teach us, O God, in this
season of approaching holiday
that we who are so used to
receiving the bounty of others
are missing the most of life if
we do not learn the Joy of
giving. We make our friends
happier by giving, and happy
friends are themselves the
best of God's gifts.

W. E. B. Du Bois

I am a Christmas contradiction.
I'm up with excitement and then
down with disappointment. I'm up
with anticipation and then down
with depression. . . . I'm on my sea-
sonal seesaw. My teeter-totter
partner is my own Currier-and-Ives
expectations. . . . I don't know
why I can't remember, from one
season to the next, that Currier
and Ives is an unattainable height.

Patsy Clairmont

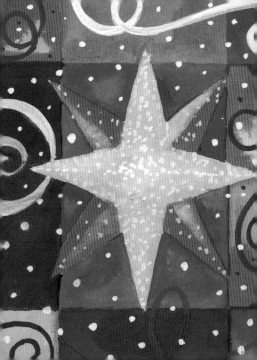

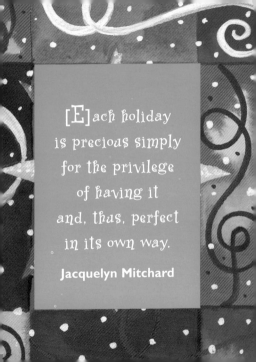

[E]ach holiday
is precious simply
for the privilege
of having it
and, thus, perfect
in its own way.

Jacquelyn Mitchard

During the Christmas season
all people the world over are looking
for miracles ... World-weary souls
soften and become open windows
through which miraculous deeds
can fly and happen upon the unwary,
who might shut them out at
other times of the year.

Jamie C. Miller, Laura Lewis,
and Jennifer Basye Sander

What will your children remember about Christmas Day, when it finally arrives? . . . Years from now, as adults, they will catch a glimpse of something, hear a snatch of song, smell food cooking . . . and today will return to them in a flood of memory.

Bishop Edmond Lee Browning

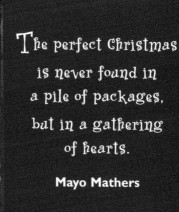

The perfect Christmas
is never found in
a pile of packages,
but in a gathering
of hearts.

Mayo Mathers

Nobody sees Santa Claus, but that is no sign that there is no Santa Claus. The most real things in the world are those that neither children nor men can see.

Francis P. Church

Like the Magi,
we have sought the Star. . . .
We ponder it
and wonder at it.
The Star that fills our
imaginations has never been
reduced to simplicity.
It shines still.

Jeanne K. Hanson

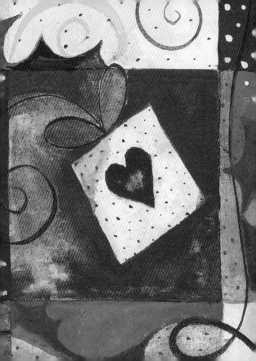

We have been miseducated
about gift-giving.
We believe gifts must always
bear a price tag or be given
for a particular reason. . . .
The real joy in giving comes
when we give what we
have spontaneously, . . .

Iyanla Vanzant

[A]sk yourself what are the most important things you can give . . . If I could create a perfect shopping list, it would include presents that you will never find in a shopping center or mail-order catalog.

Wayne W. Dyer

The holidays we observe
at this time of year
celebrate miraculous events.
Because we know these stories
of the miraculous, we long
for a miracle in our lives most
keenly in these weeks. . . .
The perception of miracle
in your life is up to you.

Barbara Cawthorne Crafton

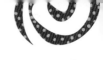

Many people nowadays say that Christmas is for children . . . Perhaps they have misplaced their sense of wonder . . . My memories cover six decades, and I am again a little child at Christmas.

Ferrol Sams

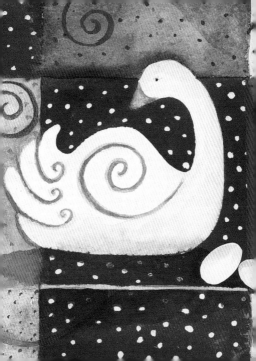

I drift along into the holidays—let them overtake me unexpectedly—waking up some fine morning and suddenly saying to myself: "Why, this is Christmas Day!"

David Grayson

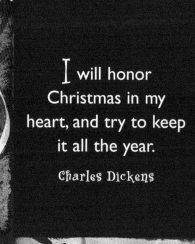

I will honor Christmas in my heart, and try to keep it all the year.

Charles Dickens

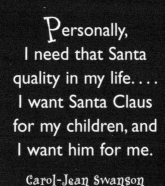

Personally,
I need that Santa
quality in my life....
I want Santa Claus
for my children, and
I want him for me.

Carol-Jean Swanson

As a child I was faced with a phenomenon requiring explanation. I hung up at the end of my bed an empty stocking, which in the morning became a full stocking. I had done nothing to produce the things that filled it. I had not worked for them, or made them or helped to make them. I had

not even been good—
far from it. And the explanation was that a certain being
whom people called Santa
Claus was benevolently
disposed towards me. . . .
And, as I say, I believe it still.

G. K. Chesterton

Why am I having
24 people to dinner?
Why am I baking nine
dozen Christmas cookies?
Why indeed? Christmas is
as good a time as any
to practice the art of
enlightened selfishness.

Jo Coudert

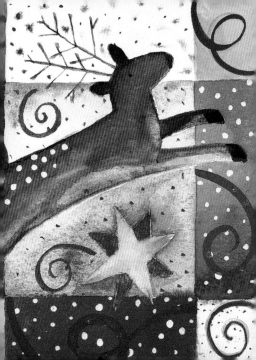

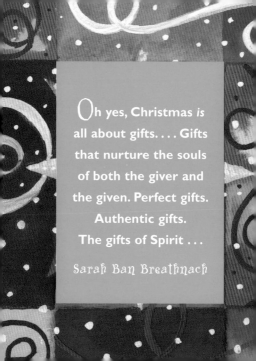

Oh yes, Christmas *is* all about gifts.... Gifts that nurture the souls of both the giver and the given. Perfect gifts. Authentic gifts. The gifts of Spirit ...

Sarah Ban Breathnach

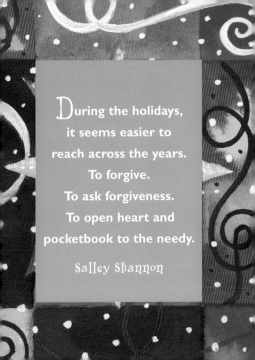

During the holidays,
it seems easier to
reach across the years.
To forgive.
To ask forgiveness.
To open heart and
pocketbook to the needy.

Salley Shannon

Even to those who say that Christmas is a myth, just the possibility of it, the fact that millions upon millions have believed it, gives the feast its ultimate meaning. Voltaire is supposed to have said that if God did not exist he would have to be invented. But who could have invented Christmas?

John Cogley

I've since discovered that there's solace to be found in observing the rituals of joy when you are alone, afraid or grieving. To inhale the scent of pine boughs or light the candles is to savour a heritage of hope.

Rona Maynard

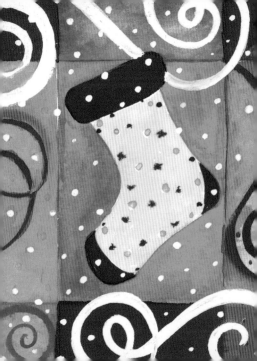

[G]iving liberates
the soul of the giver. . . .
Since time is the one
immaterial object which we
cannot influence—neither
speed up nor slow down,
add to nor diminish—
it is an imponderably
valuable gift.

Maya Angelou

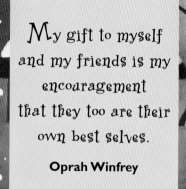

My gift to myself and my friends is my encouragement that they too are their own best selves.

Oprah Winfrey

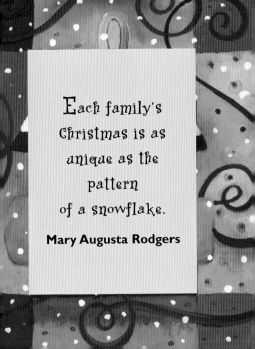

Each family's
Christmas is as
unique as the
pattern
of a snowflake.

Mary Augusta Rodgers

I made myself
a resolution for holidays
to come—one I'd like to pass
on: Have yourself a merry
little Christmas. And, honey,
just do what you can.

Gerri Hirshey

"A Merry Christmas
to us all, my dears.
God bless us!"
"God bless us every one!"
said Tiny Tim,
the last of all.

Charles Dickens,
A Christmas Carol

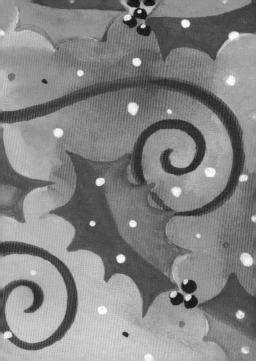

But neither prophets nor angels are absolutely essential to a miracle. Rewards . . . may come at the hands of the most unlikely individuals, and the most mundane of gifts may waken wonder in the eyes of a small boy.

Hartley F. Dailey

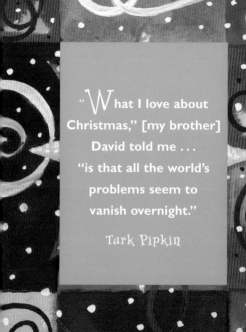

"What I love about Christmas," [my brother] David told me . . . "is that all the world's problems seem to vanish overnight."

Turk Pipkin

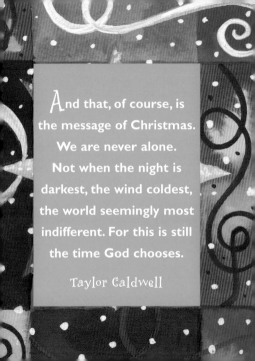

And that, of course, is the message of Christmas. We are never alone. Not when the night is darkest, the wind coldest, the world seemingly most indifferent. For this is still the time God chooses.

Taylor Caldwell

The best kind
of adjectives I use to
describe Christmas,
I also use to define my
life—simplicity, values,
family, home, and
old-fashioned kinds
of things.

Thomas Kinkade

And, always,
remember the guiding
principle of Christmas:
More is better.
And this doesn't
mean presents.
More love.
More kindness. More hope.

Mary Seehafer Sears

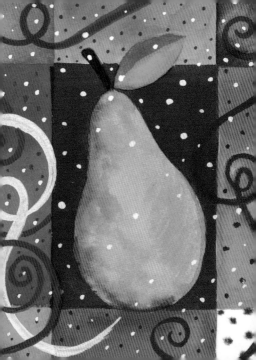

There's a lifelong glory to the Christmas season, from wide-eyed childhood to old age. It's an inexpressible glory. Keep it that way always.

Norman Vincent Peale

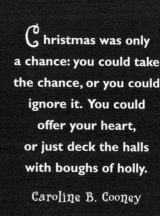

Christmas was only
a chance: you could take
the chance, or you could
ignore it. You could
offer your heart,
or just deck the halls
with boughs of holly.

Caroline B. Cooney

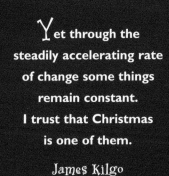

Yet through the steadily accelerating rate of change some things remain constant. I trust that Christmas is one of them.

James Kilgo

People always complain that Christmas starts too soon—that the tinsel is up in the stores right after Halloween . . . But a bigger problem, I think, is that Christmas doesn't last long enough.

Bill McKibben

[T]he Christmas
spirit comes to us
most abundantly
as we give
ourselves to others.

Sandi Schureman

This Christmas
will be our best ever,
because we are
determined to turn
back to the days when
it was just us, happy
to be together, grateful
for the love we share.

Nikki Giovanni

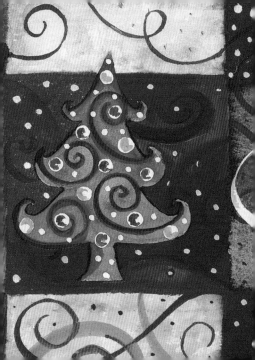

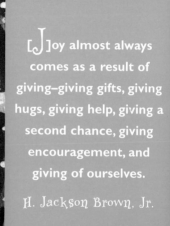

[J]oy almost always comes as a result of giving—giving gifts, giving hugs, giving help, giving a second chance, giving encouragement, and giving of ourselves.

H. Jackson Brown, Jr.

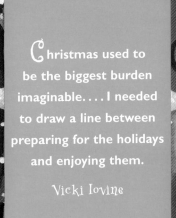

Christmas used to
be the biggest burden
imaginable....I needed
to draw a line between
preparing for the holidays
and enjoying them.

Vicki Iovine

The magi, as you
know, were wise men—
wonderfully wise men . . .
They invented the art
of giving Christmas
presents.

O. Henry

Christmas is the
mainstay of my year
because tradition is
the mainstay of my life.
It keeps me whole.

Anna Quindlen

[T]he gift
of a loving heart
at Christmas
is truly the
greatest gift of all.

Olivia Pratt

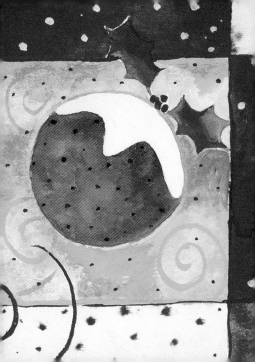

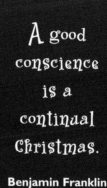

A good
conscience
is a
continual
Christmas.

Benjamin Franklin

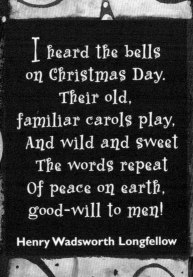

I heard the bells
on Christmas Day.
Their old,
familiar carols play,
And wild and sweet
The words repeat
Of peace on earth,
good-will to men!

Henry Wadsworth Longfellow

When you get right
down to it, all we ever
really needed to know
about how to live we
learned from Santa Claus:
Believe in yourself
and others will too.

Laura B. Randolph

The true meaning
of Christmas is expressed
in the sharing of one's
graces in a world in
which it is so easy
to become callous,
insensitive, and hard.

Howard Thurman

Families are great,
and mine is nearly perfect.
But when the holidays
come, it's only natural—
and traditional—to want
to reach out and
hug a stranger.

Barbara Ehrenreich

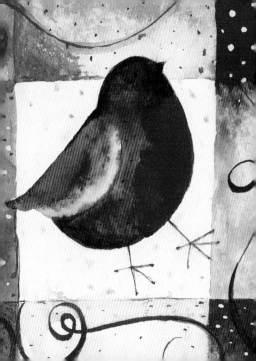

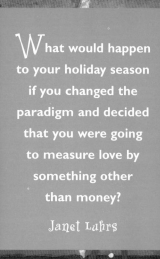

What would happen to your holiday season if you changed the paradigm and decided that you were going to measure love by something other than money?

Janet Luhrs

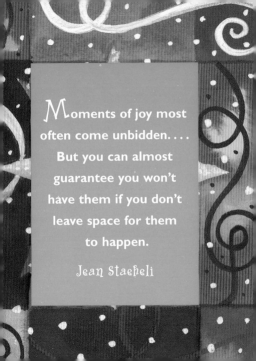

Moments of joy most often come unbidden. . . . But you can almost guarantee you won't have them if you don't leave space for them to happen.

Jean Staeheli

I do hope
your Christmas has . . .
a little touch
of Eternity in among
the rush and pitter
patter and all.

Evelyn Underhill

More than any other
holiday, Christmas opens
the floodgates of memory.

Norman M. Lobsenz

I wish you all
a Merry Christmas!
I wish us all a world as kind
as a child can imagine it!

Dorothy Thompson

Remember that even the most grown-up of grown-ups likes to feel like a kid at Christmas.

Dawn Raffel

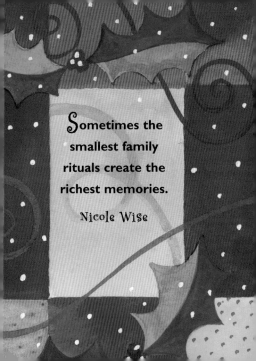

Sometimes the smallest family rituals create the richest memories.

Nicole Wise

This season we have
the opportunity to let
ourselves feel the meaning
of peace—peace within
and peace with the world.

Anne Wilson Schaef

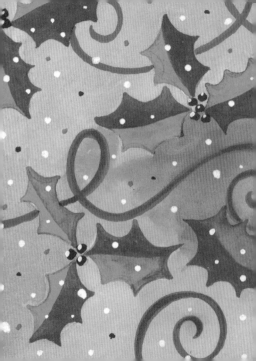